Published by Crown Publishers

Contents

1000 calorie diet?

The 1000 calorie diet has become increasingly popular over the past few years as a means of losing weight, and it's no surprise why. It's a simple and effective way to reduce your calorie intake and can result in fast weight loss. But is it really as safe and effective as it seems? The 1000 calorie diet is a very low calorie diet, so it should be approached with caution. If you decide to try it, it's important to do so under the supervision of a doctor or dietitian. This diet can be hard to follow, and it's important to make sure you're getting enough essential nutrients. The 1000 calorie diet is based on the idea that reducing your calorie intake will lead to a decrease in body fat. It's important to note, however, that this diet is not suitable for everyone. People with certain medical conditions, such as diabetes or heart disease, should not attempt this diet without medical supervision. Additionally, pregnant or breastfeeding women should not follow this diet. The 1000 calorie diet is restrictive, so it can be difficult to stick to for the long-term. It's important to be aware of the potential side effects, such as fatigue, lightheadedness, and dizziness. You may also be at risk for nutrient deficiencies, so it's important to take a daily multivitamin and pay close attention to the foods you're eating. In addition to reducing your calorie intake, it's important to make sure you're getting enough physical activity. Exercise can help to speed up weight loss and improve overall health. It's important to find activities that you enjoy, such as walking, biking, swimming, or running, and stick to them. Although the 1000 calorie diet can be an effective way to lose weight, it's important to approach it with caution. It's important to remember that this diet is not suitable for everyone, and it can be difficult to stick to for the long-term. Additionally, it's important to make sure you're getting enough essential nutrients and physical activity. If you decide to try the 1000 calorie diet, it's important to do so under the supervision of a doctor or dietitian.

Losing Weight With The 1000 Calorie Diet?

Losing weight with the 1000 calorie diet is a popular way to quickly shed unwanted pounds. But it is also a commitment that you must be willing to make in order to see the results you desire. Not only is it a calorie-restricted diet, but it also requires discipline and dedication to stick to it.

The 1000 calorie diet is designed to reduce your overall calorie intake by 500-1000 calories per day in order to achieve weight loss. It is important to note that this is not a diet to be followed for more than a few weeks at a time as it can be dangerous if followed for extended periods without medical supervision.

When starting out on a 1000 calorie diet, it is important to understand that it is necessary to eat a variety of healthy, nutrient-dense foods. Eating foods such as lean proteins, complex carbohydrates, healthy fats, fruits, and vegetables is essential in order to get the nutrients your body needs. Eating processed foods, sugary drinks, and high-calorie snacks should be avoided as they provide empty calories and will not help you reach your weight loss goals.

It is also important to understand that in order for a 1000 calorie diet to be successful, physical activity must be incorporated. This does not have to be intense exercise, but rather something that will increase your heart rate and help to burn extra calories such as walking, running, biking, swimming, or any other type of aerobic exercise.

One of the benefits of a 1000 calorie diet is that it can be adjusted to fit your lifestyle and can be customized to meet your individual needs. For example, if you have a busy lifestyle, you can adjust the diet to include snacks that are low in calories but still provide the nutrients your body needs. Another way to adjust the diet is to include more fiber-rich foods such as fruits and vegetables, as fiber helps to keep you full for longer.

In conclusion, the 1000 calorie diet can be an effective way to lose weight if done correctly. However, it is important to be aware of the potential risks and to seek advice from a medical professional if needed. Additionally, it is important to ensure that you are getting the nutrients your body needs and that you are incorporating physical activity in order to reach your weight loss goals. With the right plan and dedication, the 1000 calorie diet can help you achieve your weight loss goals.

The 1000 Calorie Diet: The Secret To Rapid Weight Loss

Hey you!

Yes you, reading this article.

I know what you're thinking...

1000 calories per day.

"Man if I just went on a 1000 calorie diet, I would lose weight so fucking fast."

"I could lose like 50 pounds in 6 weeks if I just ate 1000 calories per day."

Oh but my friend, I hate to burst your bubble.

A lot of people like the idea of 1000 calories a day.

It's a nice round number and it's associated with rapid fat loss.

Problem is, it doesn't always work in the way most people intend it to.

The#1 problem with a 1000 calorie diet

Does eating 1000 calories per day work?

Yes, if you've spent your whole life eating 3000+ calories per day, then dropping to 1000 calories per day is going to result in weight loss.

Nothing mind blowing there.

And let's put aside issues like muscle loss and not getting enough nutrients.

The #1 problem with doing a 1000 calorie per day diet, above all else, is adherence.

In other words, people can't stick with this shit long term.

90% of people who do 1000 calorie diets are in the "I want to lose weight as fast as possible" mindset.

This means they don't give a fuck about anything else but bringing the scale down.

But deep down these people know that they're just looking for a magic bullet solution to fix their shitty habits.

Eating 1000 calories a day will likely help you lose weight, but it's damn near impossible to maintain.

Focus on fixing your habits. Focus on finding a sustainable way to create a calorie deficit.

But no wants to hear that.

That advice is just way too logical

Who should eat 1000 calories a day?

While I'm not a huge fan of telling people to eat 1000 calories a day, there are a few groups of people who would benefit from doing it.

Group 1: Short people weight loss

Group 2: People with 30+ pounds to lose

Group 3: People who want to eat a lot on the weekend and still lose weight

And this isn't just mindlessly following a 1000 calorie diet. It's eating 1000 calories per day in context of your goals and lifestyle.

Group 1: Shorter people who don't weigh a lot

Who should use this: People on the shorter side and weigh 120 pounds and below.

I ain't hating on short people.

But truth is, shorter people just can't eat as much, especially if they aren't active.

Reality is, if you're 5'1" and weigh 110 pounds, then yes, you'll likely need to eat as little as 1000 calories if you want to lose weight.

That's just the truth.

But if you're on the shorter side, you need to first ask yourself: Do I even need to lose weight?

Using the same example, if you are 5'1" and weigh 105 pounds, is losing weight really the right move?

Everyone I encounter who wants to lose weight at this height and weight range just wants to "look better" (vague as fuck, I know).

But looking better doesn't always equal losing weight.

In a lot of these cases, these people would do better focusing on getting stronger and building muscle.

Building more muscle will also let you eat more food.

The big issue here is that these people have spent all of their lives obsessed with the scale.

So when I tell them to pay less attention to the scale, start lifting heavy weights, and eat more, they tell me to fuck off.

(Okay, they don't tell me to fuck off, but they don't listen to me).

If your goal is to "look better," then explore the possibility that maybe losing weight isn't the answer and maybe you just need to build muscle and strength. 2

Group 2: People with 30+ pounds to lose

Who should use this: People with 30+ pounds to lose

With Group 2, we have people with a lot for weight to lose (30+ pounds).

The more you weigh, the longer you can stay on a 1000 calorie per day diet without any crazy negative effects.

Your body can survive longer because you have more body fat to fuel it.

So someone with 30+ pounds to lose can likely stay on a 1000 calorie diet for a few weeks without negative effects.

But I'm not going to recommend that since a few weeks is just too unrealistic.

Here's my protocol for people with a lot of weight to lose and want to try a 1000 calorie diet:

If you have 30+ pounds to lose, you can eat 1000 calories per day for a week.

After the week, transition to a more sustainable diet – one where your daily calorie intake is about 10-12x your bodyweight in pounds.

Very simple.

Don't fuck this up.

Knowing people, they will fuck it up.

But man, just follow the tip I just gave.

It's 2 steps:

Step 1: Eat 1000 calories for a week.

Step 2: After the one week, set your daily calorie intake to daily calorie intake to 10-12x your bodyweight in pounds.

I swear to fucking shit, if someone leaves a comment asking me if they can do this for more than a week, I will punch a goldfish.

Think of the 1000 calorie week as a "jumpstart" to your weight loss.

You could probably do it longer, but most people just can't maintain such a large deficit.

This is not a crash diet.

This is not a quick fix or hack.

It's a jumpstart.

Some people lose up to 15 pounds in a single week.

But remember that the majority will be water weight which is is good to lose as well.

Once you transition to a more sustainable and realistic diet like I said in Step 2, your weight loss will taper off eventually into the realm of 1-2 pounds per week.

Group 3: People who want to eat a lot on the weekend and still lose weight

Who should use this: People who want to eat a crap ton of food on the weekend and still lose weight.

This is is exactly what I recommend you to do if you know you're going to go out on the weekend and drown in an orgy of beer, burgers, and fries.

Here's the 3-step process to pulling this off:

Step 1: 1-2 days out of the week, eat just 1000 calories. I recommend eating just one meal during this day to make the meal more filling. You can do 2-3 meals but then each meal becomes tiny as balls. Also make this day a high protein, low carb, low fat day. That means 90% of your calories should be pure protein. I recommend a lot of lean meat and veggies.

Step 2: On the day you know you're going to be eating a lot, enjoy yourself. Don't be stupid and binge but there's no need to count calories. Still make sure to get plenty of protein.

Step 3: On all other days of the week, follow a more conventional diet where your daily calorie intake is around 10-12x your bodyweight in pounds.

By inserting one or two 1000 calorie days during the week, you've effectively created a "buffer" for you to enjoy yourself on the weekend and still lose weight.

When it comes to weight loss, your overall weekly calories matter more than your exact daily calorie intake.

You can eat in a surplus on one day, but as long as you course correct that somewhere else during the week, you'll usually be fine.

1,000-Calorie Diet Sample Menu

Fill your 1000-calorie diet menu with nutrient-rich veggies.

A 1,000-calorie diet is a low-calorie diet typically used for women to promote weight loss. However, this diet falls below the minimum recommended calorie intake requirements for good health and may not be an adequate source of nutrients, which may lead to deficiencies. Given the limitations of the diet, including nutrient-rich foods is an important aspect of a 1,000-calorie diet plan. Always consult your doctor before making any changes to your diet -- especially for such a low-calorie diet, which should only be followed under ongoing medical supervision.

1,000-Calorie Diet Basics

When following a low-calorie diet such as the 1,000-calorie diet, you have very little room for extras and indulgences, so you want to make sure your food choices are rich in nutrients and low in calories to get the most nutrition out of every bite. That means filling your plate with fruits and vegetables, lean sources of protein, whole grains, low-fat or nonfat dairy and healthy fats. Fitting in most of the food groups at each meal can help make sure you get enough nutrients.

To stay energized and satisfied, be sure to eat at regular intervals throughout the day, every three to four hours, which means three 300-calorie meals and one 100-calorie snack. Most importantly, don't skip meals to save calories or hasten your weight loss because you may sabotage your efforts by creating an intense hunger that leads to overeating.

Sample Menu: Breakfast

Start the day right with a healthy and filling breakfast. A good sample meal might include 1/2 cup of nonfat cottage cheese with a small banana and a slice of whole-wheat toast with 2 teaspoons of peanut butter for about 300 calories. You might also enjoy a warm bowl of oatmeal filled with 1 cup of cooked oatmeal, 3/4 cup of fresh blueberries and 4 chopped walnut halves with 1 cup of nonfat milk or nondairy alternative such as soy milk, which has 282 calories. Those with limited time for breakfast in the morning can drink a smoothie you make on-the-go consisting of 6 ounces of nonfat plain Greek yogurt, 1 cup of diced mango and 1 tablespoon of almond butter for 318 calories.

Sample Menu: Lunch

Fill your lunch with low-calorie fruits and veggies to keep hunger away in the afternoon. A good lunch might include 2 cups of mixed greens topped with 2 ounces of grilled chicken breast, 1/4 cup of kidney beans, and 2 tablespoons of low-fat salad dressing with 1 cup of cubed cantaloupe and 6 ounces of nonfat Greek yogurt for 322 calories. Or, fill half a whole-wheat pita with 2 tablespoons of hummus, lettuce and shredded carrot, and serve it with 1 cup of sliced cucumbers, a small orange and 1 ounce of low-fat cheese, which has 295 calories. Two-ounces of water-packed canned tuna mixed with 1 tablespoon of low-fat mayonnaise served with 10 whole-grain crackers with 1 cup of sliced carrots and celery sticks and two plums for 315 calories also makes a healthy lunch option on your 1,000-calorie diet plan.

Sample Menu: Dinner

End your day on a good note with a nutrient-rich dinner such as 3 ounces of grilled salmon with 1/2 cup of roasted sweet potatoes and 2 cups of steamed broccoli and cauliflower, which has 295 calories. A veggie stir-fry made with 1 cup of sliced carrots, celery, onions and bok choy with 1/2 cup of tofu sauteed in 1 teaspoon of vegetable oil and served with 1/2 cup of cooked brown rice also makes a healthy dinner meal at 290 calories. A 2-ounce turkey burger on a whole-wheat hamburger bun with 1 cup of mixed greens topped with 2 tablespoons of low-fat salad dressing makes another healthy dinner option with 300 calories.

Snack Ideas

Snacks tide you over in between meals, so make them filling and healthy. For 100 calories, try one of these: 2 cups of mixed greens topped with 2 tablespoons of low-fat salad dressing; 14 almonds; a small apple with 1 ounce of low-fat cheese; one container of nonfat Greek yogurt; 2 tablespoons of hummus with 2 cups of sliced peppers, cucumbers and carrots or 1/2 cup of whole-grain unsweetened cereal with 1/2 cup of nonfat milk or milk alternative.

1000 Calorie Diet Plan – Is It Good For Weight Loss?

A 1000 calorie diet plan or a low-calorie diet plan is used for rapid weight loss. The rationale behind the 1000 calorie diet plan is that a drastic reduction in calorie intake results in weight loss with little or no physical activity. In this diet plan, you are allowed to consume limited carbohydrates, more low-calorie fruits and vegetables, and lean proteins. A low-calorie diet is effective in reducing body weight by an average of 8%, but this is a short-term approach.

Caution: Consult a doctor or a nutritionist before going on this diet as it involves a drastic reduction in calorie intake.

The 1000 Calorie Diet Chart (Sample Plan)

This 1000 calorie diet chart is a sample menu that can be followed by anyone who wants to lose weight drastically. The plan may vary based on your weight and physical activity. Consult a doctor or a dietitian to adjust it according to your body's requirements.

Variation 1

MEAL WHAT TO EAT CALORIES

Early Morning Apple cider vinegar and warm water 6

Breakfast 2 boiled egg whites and a bowl of fruit 86

Pre-Lunch 100 g of low-fat yogurt 154

Lunch Lettuce taco with yogurt sauce 351

Post-Lunch 1 bowl of watermelon 46

Evening Snack Green tea and 2 digestive biscuits 142

Dinner Vegan salads with fat-free salad dressing 221

Total Calorie Intake – 1008

Useful Tip – You can also have green tea in the morning instead of a detox drink. Green tea has 0 calories. A study done on mice states that it is rich in the antioxidant epigallocatechin gallate (EGCG) that has an anti-obesity effect.

Variation 2

MEAL WHAT TO EAT CALORIES

Early Morning Honey, lemon juice, and warm water 70

Breakfast Oatmeal with strawberries 101

Pre-Lunch Green tea 0

Lunch Cabbage soup and 100 g low-fat yogurt 227

Post-Lunch 1 peach and 1 orange 98

Evening Snack Green tea and 2 digestive biscuits 142

Dinner 1 bowl of boiled lentils with stir-fried French beans, capsicum, and peas with a dash of chopped garlic 386

Total Calorie Intake – 1024

Variation 3

MEAL WHAT TO EAT CALORIES

Early Morning Veggie smoothie made of 1 carrot, 1 tomato, 1 cucumber, and a handful of spinach 98

Breakfast Soy milk, 1 slice of multigrain bread, and 2 boiled egg whites OR Soy milk and 1 banana 157 OR 159

Pre- Lunch 1 glass buttermilk (if following a non-vegan diet) OR 1 glass watermelon and kiwi juice 40 OR 91

Lunch Chicken clear soup with veggies OR Roasted veggies with 100 g yogurt 187 OR 152

Post-Lunch 1 pear and 1 orange 143

Evening Snack Green tea and 2 digestive biscuits 142

Dinner Baked fish and 100g yogurt OR Vegetable clear soup (cabbage, onion, garlic, carrot) with 2 slices of whole wheat bread. 296 OR 265

Total Calorie Intake – 1050

Video – Expert Speaks About 1000 Calorie Diet

In this video, StyleCraze's in-house diet expert speaks about the 1000-calorie diet. She provides a complete picture of what is good for dieters who want to try the 1000-calorie diet. Watch this video to know more:

What To Eat

The selection of foods for a 1000-calorie diet should be done carefully to create a healthy menu that will get you the desired results.

• The 1000-calorie diet plan should incorporate foods that are rich in vitamin B, proteins, and fiber, normally found in wheat foods and enzymes.

- The diet demands a reduction in whole food types, like carbs or trans fats, as your body requires nutrition to improve overall health.

- Calcium can be included by taking low-fat milk and green vegetables. Do not ignore fruits and vegetables.

- Fruits like oranges, cantaloupes, kiwi, pears, strawberries, and numerous other berries that offer minimal calories can be used in salads.

- Green veggies like spinach, celery, zucchini, broccoli, and artichokes are rich in vitamins and minerals besides being low-calorie ingredients.

• A single portion of cabbage contains just 35 calories but is pretty rich in nutritional fiber.

• Apart from this, vegetables like cucumber, celery, and eco-friendly peppers have high water content.

What Not To Eat

Here is the list of foods you should absolutely avoid when you are on the 1000-calorie diet:

- Fats And Oils – Coconut oil, groundnut oil, walnut oil, palm oil, avocado oil, lard, and other animal fat oil, butter, peanut butter, almond butter, cashew butter, cheese, cream cheese, and ghee.

- Seeds And Nuts – Hazelnuts, cashew nuts, watermelon seeds, walnuts, pine nuts, desiccated coconut, peanuts, Brazil nuts, pistachio, and chia seeds.

- Dry Fruits – Dates, prunes, dried currants, apricots, figs, and cranberries.

- Fruits, Veggies, And Legumes – Avocado, mango, litchi, chiku, custard apple, potato, corn, lima beans, and soybeans.

- Proteins – Beef, pork, lamb, and tofu.

Grocery List

Before creating a 1000-calorie diet plan, you need to make your kitchen healthy. Plan your grocery list beforehand. Here is a list of items that you need to stock up on before you start this diet:

• As it is a low-carb plan, limit buying any grains.

• Seafood, fish, and lean protein like chicken breast.

• Pulses and legumes.

• Seasonal colorful fruits and vegetables.

• Low-fat milk and dairy products.

• Spices and condiments to boost your metabolism.

The 1000 Calorie Diet Recipe

You can control your calorie intake per day, but that does not mean you have to eat boring food. Make your meals exciting and tasty using seasonal veggies, meat, and spices available in the supermarket, but with a twist.

1. Lettuce Taco With Yogurt Sauce

What You Need

• 2 fresh lettuce leaves

• 1/2 cucumber

• 1/2 cucumber

- 1/2 red and yellow bell peppers

- 1 tomato

- 1/2 skinless chicken breast

- 1/2 tablespoon lemon juice

- 1/2 jalapeno

- 100 g yogurt

- A handful of cilantro

- 1 teaspoon chili flakes

- A pinch of salt

- A pinch of pepper

How To Prepare

1. Season the skinless chicken breast with salt and pepper and boil it.

2. Shred the boiled chicken breast.

3. Grate the cucumber.

4. Julienne the bell peppers and slice the tomato.

5. Slice the jalapeno.

6. Take 100 g yogurt in a medium-sized bowl.

7. Add the grated cucumber, a pinch of salt, and chili flakes. Mix well.

8. Wash the lettuce leaves.

9. Place the sliced tomatoes on the lettuce leaves.

10. Add the shredded chicken.

11. Add a little salt and black pepper if needed.

12. Add the bell peppers and jalapenos.

13. Put a generous dollop of yogurt sauce on top.

14. Finally, add a few cilantro/coriander leaves.

Vegetarian Alternative

If you are a vegetarian, instead of chicken, you can add carrots, stir-fried broccoli florets, and button mushrooms.

Benefits

• The skinless chicken breast is low in calories and a good source of protein, iron, and polyunsaturated fat (3).

• Cucumbers are super low in calories. They are good sources of vitamins C and A, magnesium, iron, calcium, and potassium (4).

• The colorful bell peppers are rich in vitamins C and A, potassium, dietary fiber, and minerals, such as magnesium, potassium, and iron.

• Lettuce leaves are low in calories and a good source of vitamins A and C, iron, calcium, magnesium, and potassium.

• Yogurt is a good source of good gut bacteria that help in digestion.

2. Delicious Vegan Ribbons Salad

What You Need

- 1 zucchini

- 1 carrot

- 1 tomato

- A handful of spinach

- 1 tablespoon of sesame oil

- Juice of half a lemon

- A few coriander leaves

- A pinch of salt and black pepper

How To Prepare

1. Peel the zucchini and carrot into thin ribbons.

2. Julienne the tomato.

3. Roughly chop a handful of spinach.

4. Make the salad dressing by adding sesame oil and lemon juice in a separate bowl and beating the mixture.

5. Add a little salt and pepper to the salad dressing. Mix well.

6. Add the salad dressing to the veggies.

7. Mix well to coat the dressing evenly on the veggies.

8. Garnish with coriander leaves.

Non-Vegetarian Alternative

You can add 2-3 thin slices of turkey bacon to this salad.

Benefits

• Zucchini is a low-calorie food and a good source of vitamins C, B6, and A. It has a good amount of potassium, magnesium, dietary fiber, and iron.

• Carrots are very rich in vitamin A, potassium, magnesium, and dietary fiber.

• Spinach has a good amount of vitamins A, C, and B6. It is also a good source of magnesium, iron, potassium, calcium, and dietary fiber (10).

Role Of Exercise When On The 1000-Calorie Diet

Exercising is a healthy habit. However, the 1000-calorie diet is a low-calorie diet plan for you to lose weight quickly. That is why rigorous exercising is not recommended when you are on this diet. Here's what you can do:

• Go for a medium-paced walk for 30 minutes daily.

• Do some stretching exercises to improve blood circulation.

• You can try low-impact exercises that burn calories without causing any pain in the joints and muscles.

Caution:If you feel weak after exercising, consult a doctor and stop working out.

Benefits Of The 1000 Calorie Diet

• The 1000 calorie diet is considered useful when it comes to burning calories at a fast rate as it is a low-calorie diet. This diet is apt if you intend to lose a few pounds quickly or pave the way for a long-term weight loss plan.

- The sample menu of this diet plan provides good nutrition when it is well-balanced.

- This diet primarily emphasizes the consumption of fruits and vegetables as they have few calories and high content of water and fiber, which provides a feeling of fullness and prevents you from overeating.

- It is simple and easy to follow, encourages healthy eating, enables you to shed a few extra pounds, and boosts your confidence.

Side Effects Of The 1000 Calorie Diet

• As it is a low-calorie diet, it lacks certain vital nutrients that provide energy to the body.

• Due to the lack of nutrition, this diet can cause dehydration, loss in muscle mass, lack of energy, slower heart rate, hair loss, and weaker nails.

• The drastic cut in calories lowers your metabolism. A lower metabolic rate results in rapid weight gain when the caloric intake is increased in the future.

• This diet is suitable for women who have a small frame. It is not considered suitable for men. It can be potentially dangerous for people who have well-built or athletic bodies.

• Starvation is another ill effect of this diet. Exhaustion resulting from the diet can make you susceptible to injuries.

• It can cause fatigue and loss of concentration and make you moody.

• It can cause insomnia.

What Should You Follow?

Do's Don'ts

Follow the diet for not more than 10 days. Do not overeat.

Consult your doctor before following the 1000-calorie diet. Avoid alcohol and sweetened and carbonated beverages.

Go for medium-paced walks and light exercises. Do not sit in one place for too long.

Include lots of fresh fruits and veggies in your diet. Do not skip any of the meals.

Consume a good amount of proteins to build your muscle strength. Do not take stress if you have gone a little above 1000 calories one day. Skip the bowl of watermelon the next day and have a cup of green tea instead.

Drink enough water. Do not stay awake late at night.

Note: As it is a low-calorie diet plan, you must consume multivitamin and mineral supplements along with vitamin D3. Always consult a doctor before taking any supplements.

Conclusion

Though the 1000-calorie diet is an effective way to reduce weight quickly, it should be done under the guidance of a doctor or a nutritionist. A low-calorie diet plan involves balancing macronutrients with low carbs and fat and moderate protein. Your plate should be loaded with low-calorie fruits and vegetables. Starving yourself or following an imbalanced low-calorie diet will lead to more weight gain once you stop following the diet.

Expert's Answers for Readers Questions

How many pounds can you lose if you go on a 1000-calorie diet?

With a 1000-calorie diet, you can reduce up to 8% of your present weight. Every body type is different, so weight loss may vary from anywhere between 5 pounds to 10 pounds.

What lean proteins can I have while on the 1000-calorie diet?

You can have skinless chicken, turkey, fish, button mushrooms, and lentils. Avoid beans, tofu, beef, and pork.

I weigh 250 lbs and want to lose weight quickly. Can I go on the 1000-calorie diet for a month?

Depending on your body type, metabolic rate, genetics, age, and medical history, you need to follow a diet that will not harm your body in the long term. Exercising is a healthy option to start with. If you starve yourself, you will gain weight instead of losing it. Seek your doctor's advice so that your calorie intake is reduced gradually.

Can I lose weight without exercising if I am on the 1000-calorie diet?

Since the 1000-calorie diet has way lesser calories than what you should normally intake, you can pretty much do without exercising. Do some stretching and medium-paced walks to maintain your blood circulation and muscle strength.

I am a breastfeeding mother. Is the 1000-calorie diet right for me?

If you are breastfeeding, it is not advisable to go on a low-calorie diet. You should consult your doctor or dietitian to know whether you can go on a low-calorie diet so soon.

Can I have a cheat day while on the 1000-calorie diet?

Yes, you can. Make sure you eat in less portions. This will help you the next day. If you eat about 2000 calories (or more), and the next day you want to fast, that is not an option and is not recommended at all. Once a week, you can have slightly more than 1000 calories, say 1300-1400 calories. Nullify the effect by sticking to the diet and drinking green tea at least twice a day for the next two days.

Everything You Need to Know Before Trying a 1,000-Calorie-a-Day Meal Plan

Fill up on low-calorie, nutrient-rich foods on your 1,000-calorie diet plan.

Image Credit: anakopa/iStock/Getty Images

To lose weight, you need to reduce your calorie intake. But limiting your intake to 1,000 calories a day may make a diet difficult to follow over the long term and could potentially lead to nutritional deficiencies. If you're considering a 1,000-calorie diet to help you lose the weight, consult your doctor for ongoing support and guidance.

Risks and Benefits of a 1,000-Calorie Diet

At a basic level, weight loss requires a calorie deficit, meaning you eat fewer calories than you burn, according to the Mayo Clinic. It's often said that one pound of fat equals 3,500 calories and so, cutting about 500 to 1,000 calories per day would theoretically spur one to two pounds of weight loss per week. But weight loss is a little more complicated than that. For example, lowering your caloric intake too far can make your body burn fat-free mass (aka lean muscle) rather than just fat, according to a December 2018 study published in Nutrients.

In fact, loss of fat-free mass is among the major drawbacks of a 1,000-calorie diet. According to the American Academy of Family Physicians, calorie restriction usually results mostly in the loss of water weight or lean muscle, not body fat. So while you could be losing pounds on the scale, the results may not be reflected in the mirror — and they might not last.

The lack of variety in a 1000-calorie diet can lead to malnutrition, sluggishness and a slower metabolism, according to the Academy of Nutrition and Dietetics. Severely cutting calories tricks your body into thinking it is in a famine condition, causing your metabolism to drop.

A 1,000-calorie diet is most likely to result in weight loss for individuals at a high starting weight. According to UCLA Health, a diet of 1,000 calories per day or less affects your body in the same way as total starvation. When severely obese individuals in particular are restricted to a very low-calorie diet, they can lose between three to five pounds per week. However, considering the dramatic shift this regimen spurs, it should be monitored by a medical professional.

Healthy Foods for a 1,000-Calorie Diet

To maximize every bite, you need to make very smart choices on your 1,000-calorie diet plan. For health and balance, you should consider the caloric density of your foods and choose wisely.

Fill your meals with leafy vegetables and fruits. Fruits and vegetables are both low in calories and high in fiber, which can help curb your hunger. For instance, while one-quarter cup of raisins contains around 100 calories, you can eat an entire cup of grapes for the same amount of calories. A small order of french fries has more than 200 calories, while a large salad might have the same caloric density.

Although a 1,000-calorie diet is certainly low, there is still room for snacks in your daily plan. Instead of choosing potato chips, opt for air-popped popcorn or fruits and veggies.

Also consider the high-calorie beverages you may be sipping throughout the day. Trade your latte for a black coffee and turn your soda into a sparkling water.

Example 1,000-Calorie Meal Plan

Breakfast

- 2-egg omelet

- 1 cup blueberries

- 1 cup black coffee

Total (according to the USDA): about 275 calories

Morning Snack

- 3 cups plain air-popped popcorn

Total: approximately 90 calories

Lunch

- 1/2 chicken breast

- 2 cups shredded lettuce

- 1 handful cherry tomatoes

- 1 small baked sweet potato

Total: roughly 260 calories

Dinner

- 3 oz. (1 serving) salmon filet

- 1 cup boiled or steamed broccoli

- 1/2 cup brown rice

Total: 300 calories

Dessert

- 1 1/2 cup strawberries

- 1 cup chamomile tea

Total: 70 calories